Spinal Breathing Pranayama

–

Journey to Inner Space

Yogani

From The AYP Enlightenment Series

AYP Publishing

For ordering information go to:

www.advancedyogapractices.com

Library of Congress Control Number: 2006923697

Published simultaneously in:

Nashville, Tennessee, U.S.A.
and
London, England, U.K.

This title is also available in eBook format – ISBN 0-9764655-7-4
(For Adobe Reader)

ISBN 0-9764655-6-6 (Paperback)

"All the while my breath is in me,
and the spirit of God is in my nostrils…"

Job 27:3

Introduction

Spinal Breathing Pranayama is one of the most important practices in all of yoga. It can have a positive impact on our health and well-being, and in facilitating more effective functioning in every aspect of our daily life. But more than that, spinal breathing pranayama purifies and opens us to our ecstatic inner realms. To engage in this simple practice on a daily basis is to be on an exciting journey to *inner space*.

For thousands of years, methods of spinal breathing have been utilized by spiritual practitioners, and are mentioned in the ancient scriptures. Yet, the details of this practice have always been kept secret from the vast majority of the population. Now, in these rapidly changing times, there is a great need for many to have access to the means that have long been reserved for the few. No one owns this knowledge. It originates inside each of us, within our very own nervous system. We only need a few simple instructions, and the natural evolutionary processes present within us will take over, yielding marvelous results.

The Advanced Yoga Practices Enlightenment Series is an endeavor to present the most effective methods of yoga in a series of easy-to-read books that anyone can use to gain practical results immediately and over the long term. Since the AYP writings first began in 2003, we have been engaged in a fascinating experiment to see just how much can be conveyed, with much more detail included on practices than in the spiritual writings of the past. Can books provide us the specific means necessary to tread the path to enlightenment, or do we have to surrender at the feet of a *guru* to find our salvation? Well, clearly we must surrender to something, even if it is to our own innate potential to live a freer and happier life. If we are able to do that, and maintain a daily practice, then books like this one can come alive and instruct us in the ways of human spiritual transformation. If the reader is ready and the book is worthy, amazing things can happen.

While one person's name is given as the author of this book, it is actually a distillation of the efforts of thousands of practitioners over thousands of years. This is one person's attempt to simplify and make practical the spiritual methods that many have utilized throughout history. All who have gone before have my deepest gratitude, as do the many I am privileged to be in touch with in the present who continue to practice with dedication and good results.

I hope you will find this book to be a useful resource as you travel along your chosen path.

Practice wisely, and enjoy!

Table of Contents

Chapter 1 – Breath and the Life Force

Breath is life. It sustains us and it is an expression of the life force within us. The fact that we are breathing is an affirmation of life. It means we want to be here. It means we want to be doing something here. But what?

So much of life is instinct. We breathe, we eat, we sleep, we become active, we procreate…

Within all of that, we are making choices about what to do with our life, going about our business – getting an education, pursuing a career, making money, raising a family, working for the things that matter to us, and so on.

All the while, something is wondering inside: "What is all this for? Why am I here? Is there something more?" We have an instinct to be asking these questions. Like breath itself, the questions are spurred through the impulse of life stirring deep within us. Indeed, the questions are an essential constituent of our life force, as essential as breathing itself.

What is this life force that sustains and animates every aspect of our existence, and spurs us on to find answers? We know that all of material existence is made up of energy. Physics tells us that all matter is empty space made to behave as solid by the polarities of energy whirling inside. All of this whirling in the vacuum of infinite space, making the appearance of matter, is according to natural laws. That is, the nature of matter is predictable, at least as far as we have been able to determine with our scientific investigations over the centuries. Likewise, when matter takes the form of living things – plants, animals and human beings – much can be predicted about the physicality of life. But there is something more manifesting in living things. The whirling energies are still there creating the appearance of matter. Yet, something more is operating to bring the matter together into an intelligent expression – an intelligent and evolving system. This something else we can call the "life force."

In the ancient teachings of yoga from India, the life force is given another name – *prana*, which means "first unit" or "first manifestation." Yoga regards the manifestation of all matter as a manifestation of prana, and therefore "intelligent." Indeed, all that exists, all that is born of energy is an expression of prana. The rocks and earth are expressions of prana. The seas are an expression of prana. The air is an expression of prana. And all of animate life is an expression of prana. In the Eastern way of thinking about it, the entire material existence is an expression of prana – the life force. And it is all imbued with an innate intelligence.

Where does prana come from? Whether we go to the spiritual teachings of the world, or to modern quantum physics, we will find a similar answer –

stillness is the source of prana, the life force that energizes the universe we experience. The stillness we speak of is of a special kind – a stillness that is filled with possibilities. It is an awareness that does not move. Yet, all that we see springs from it and is it. In the AYP writings we call it inner silence, or pure bliss consciousness. It has many names in many traditions. Whatever we call it, it is underlying all the activities of the life force, and everything we do in life.

The cultivation of inner silence in the human being is the subject of the first book in the AYP Enlightenment Series: *Deep Meditation – Pathway to Personal Freedom*. Now we are going to the next step, which is the cultivation of prana, the life force, in the human being in ways that promote the expansion of our inner potential, our inner silence.

To this end, yoga has a branch of practice called *pranayama*, which means "restraint of prana," the life force manifested as breath. So pranayama is about breathing techniques.

There are many methods of pranayama, many breathing techniques. But one stands out above all the rest. It is called *spinal breathing pranayama*. The reason it stands out is because of its effectiveness in stimulating and regulating prana within us in a way that covers the three primary objectives of all pranayama:

1. Culturing the nervous system to become a steadily improving vehicle for inner silence rising from deep meditation.

2. Awakening the nervous system to a condition of permanent *ecstatic conductivity*.

3. Increasing and balancing the flow of inner energy (prana) over the long term to facilitate a progressive and safe unfoldment of the individual toward enlightenment.

The internal dynamics of implementing these three objectives are complex. Fortunately, the practice of spinal breathing is very simple. It is like this in the successful application of any complex technology in our society. The means of control are optimized and simplified to a level where nearly anyone can efficiently take advantage of complex principles found in nature.

For example, consider a car. We hardly give it a second thought when we climb into a car and drive off to an appointment. Even as we are driving, we will be thinking about our appointment rather than the complex technology that is operating smoothly under the hood of the car, whisking us off to our chosen destination. All we have to do is press on the gas pedal and hold the steering wheel, and away we go. Simple, yes? No, not simple at all, but it has been made simple by virtue of the simplified controls that enable us to effortlessly transform a volatile substance, gasoline, into a speedy and safe ride to our appointment.

Pranayama is like that. In fact, all effective spiritual practice is like that. We can take complex principles of transformation found in the human nervous system and, with a series of simple procedures, apply these for great spiritual benefit.

In the case of spinal breathing pranayama, we are simultaneously capitalizing on numerous complex principles that are operating within our neurobiology, and we are enhancing these in a broad-based way.

As the name implies, spinal breathing involves doing something in the spine. From physiology and neurology we know that the spinal cord is the main highway of our functioning. From yoga, we know that the spinal cord is the main highway of the life force in our body. Yoga also recognizes that as we purify and open the nerves in the body, inner experiential openings occur. This is the central principle in deep meditation, where we systematically go from thinking to inner silence and come out into the body/mind with great purifying effects. This kind of process is also central in the application of spinal breathing pranayama, on the level of the breath and the body, where we are going in and cultivating the nerves in a specific and purifying way. In doing so, we are improving the ability of the subtle neurobiology to serve as a much better vehicle for inner silence brought out through deep meditation. And, with spinal breathing pranayama, we are also gradually making the body a much better conductor of the inner energies which play an increasing role as the process of human spiritual transformation advances.

Together, inner silence and the awakening of our inner energies (prana, the life force) intermingle to produce a condition of unshakable inner steadiness and ecstatic bliss. As the process refines, we find this remarkable development overflowing through our conduct in daily living and into our surroundings, gradually transforming us to become a channel of divine love flowing into the world.

Along the way we find ourselves becoming intimately familiar with our vast inner dimensions. Indeed, the journey of spiritual practices is a journey to *inner space*. This is particularly true of spinal breathing pranayama, which, in the process of setting the stage for the purification and opening of our nervous system to ecstatic bliss and the outward flow of divine love, also opens us up to a direct perception of our inner realms. Interestingly, in the process of discovering our own interior, we also discover that what is in us is also the basis of everything and everyone we see in the outside world. In coming to know ourselves, we come to know all that is around us as an expression of our own inner awareness and inner space.

While all this may seem an interesting theory, we are not here to discuss theory and philosophy much in this book. We are here to provide the means for direct experience of the things we are talking about.

So let's move on and talk about how to do spinal breathing pranayama, and also take a look at the specifics of what we may find in the way of resulting experiences.

Chapter 2 – Spinal Breathing Pranayama

We are all wired for enlightenment. We are all wired to be illuminated from within. It is only a matter of purifying the wiring, our nervous system, to know the truth of this. A primary means by which our nervous system can become purified is through spinal breathing pranayama. It is a mechanical process involving breath, attention and a few other simple components. As we engage in the practice, we will be brought in touch with our own inner anatomy, and begin to purify it step-by-step with each day of practice. The scenery we will see along the way will be dazzling at times, dull at other times, and perhaps even stuck at yet other times. But, all the while we will be traveling forward, if we keep up our daily practice.

For those who are reading this book before learning deep meditation, do keep in mind that with spinal breathing, we are preparing for deep meditation. Spinal breathing is a powerful practice. But, alone, it is not enough to complete the illumination we are talking about here. With spinal breathing we will journey to inner space. And with the addition of deep meditation immediately after our spinal breathing we will *become* inner space.

How to do Spinal Breathing

If we can breathe, think and visualize, we can do spinal breathing. Only one other skill is necessary – the ability to form a daily habit. It is not difficult. So let's begin…

We start by sitting comfortably with back support with our eyes closed. No particular posture is required. The main thing is to be comfortable and reasonably upright. We can be in a chair or sitting on the bed.

Then we just begin to notice our breathing – easily in and then easily back out. Spinal breathing is done through the nose with mouth closed. We do not use alternate nostril breathing with the fingers in this style of pranayama. If the nose is obstructed so as to make nose breathing uncomfortable, then we can breathe through our mouth. Now we will do two things.

First, we slow down our breathing in a comfortable way – no straining. We just take it to the slowest comfortable pace we can. As part of this we breathe deeper, drawing more air in and expelling more air out than we do in normal breathing. We just breathe slower and deeper, keeping comfort well in hand. No heroics are necessary. Got it? Good.

Second, we imagine a tiny nerve, like a little tube the size of a thread running from our perineum all the way up to the center of our brow. The perineum is the place underneath, between the genitals and the anus – we also call it the *root*. The center of the brow is the point between the eyebrows – sometimes it is called the *third eye*. The tiny nerve that goes between the root and the brow is called the *spinal nerve*. Between the root and the brow, the spinal nerve goes up the center of the spine to the center of the head and turns forward to the brow, like that.

What we do in spinal breathing is trace the spinal nerve with our attention as we breathe. We go up from the root to the brow on inhalation, and down from the brow to the root on exhalation. This we do over and over again for as long as we are practicing spinal breathing.

In the beginning, we are visualizing the spinal nerve and tracing it with our slow deep breathing. As our practice develops, visualization will give way to direct perception of the spinal nerve. More on that later. Until then, we will visualize, and this will be our means for awakening and enlivening the main highway of our nervous system.

If during our journey up and down the spinal nerve during slow deep breathing, we find our attention off into internal or external experiences, sensations or other stimuli, then we just easily go back to our practice of slow deep breathing up and down the spinal nerve. It is normal to lose track of what we are doing and be off into other sensations, thoughts and feelings. When we do, we just simply re-engage the process of spinal breathing again. When we realize we are off it, we just easily come back.

If we have some difficulty visualizing and tracing the spinal nerve as a tiny thread or tube, then it is perfectly all right to follow the spinal column in a less specific way. Over time, we will find more definition in our practice. There is no need to strain or struggle in our visualization. The main thing is that we end up at the brow at the completion of inhalation and at the root at the completion of exhalation. How we get back and forth is less important than traveling from one end to the other without strain during our slow deep breathing. In time, it all comes together.

Tracing the spinal nerve with slow deep breathing is the technique of spinal breathing pranayama. And when we drift off from it, we just easily come back. That is part of the practice also. No strain and no fuss. Very simple, yes? There are several more aspects that will be added later. But before we do that, let's cover a few practical matters and get some experience under our belt.

When and Where to do Spinal Breathing

The best benefits of spinal breathing will be found in keeping up a twice-daily practice session. The ideal time to do it is before the morning and evening meal. There is flexibility on this according to one's schedule. Doing pranayama on an empty stomach is preferred. It will be your choice. It is suggested to start with five minutes of spinal breathing at each sitting, followed by meditation. AYP deep meditation is recommended. If another form of meditation has been in use already with good results, it will be okay to use that method of meditation instead. But do keep in mind that by *meditation* we mean a mental technique that brings the mind and body to deep inner stillness. It is inner silence we want to be cultivating after our spinal breathing session. If no method of meditation has been in use before now, then it will be fine to sit with eyes closed and mind easy for five or ten minutes after spinal breathing before getting up. Learning an effective technique of deep meditation will be advisable so the maximum combined benefits of both spinal breathing and meditation can be achieved. The two practices go together in sequence like that – hand in glove.

Spinal breathing can be done just about anywhere. Obviously, at home on our meditation seat is the best place, but we do not always have the luxury. If we are on-the-go, spinal breathing can be done almost anywhere at the appointed time – in planes, trains, cars (not while driving!), busy waiting rooms, etc. It is a practice that can be done very discreetly, with our meditation right after. We will be sitting there with our eyes closed and no one will know that we are plumbing the depths of our cosmic realms within. Only by the happy expression on our face will they know.

Now will be a good time for you to try a spinal breathing session. Just sit comfortably and begin the practice as it has been given – very easily, with no strain. Do it for five minutes. It is okay to peek at the clock once in a while to check the time. Once you have finished, then sit for a few more minutes, relaxed, with your eyes closed.

It is a very easy practice. Even so, no doubt you will have some questions. We will cover a few of the main ones in this chapter, and many more in the next chapter.

So, go now and do a session, and then come back for some questions and answers. We'll also discuss a few additional aspects of spinal breathing practice that can be incorporated to enhance the results.

Initial Questions on Practice

Now that you have had a taste of spinal breathing, we can cover a few questions that often come up. These will cover a range, from not much happening to a lot happening – there can be some inner resistance, or no resistance at all. It can be anywhere on this scale in the first session. Everyone is different, and will experience spinal breathing according to the inner condition of their nervous system. The march of progress in spinal breathing is a process of purification and opening. This is at the heart of the journey in all spiritual practice. Purification, opening to our vast inner space, and illumination from within.

Here are three questions and answers that summarize the range of experiences we can have when starting out. In the next chapter we will delve much deeper into the relationship of practice and experiences, and how to travel the road of our inner purification to enlightenment.

This is not easy. Is it supposed to be?

Sometimes, in the beginning, there can be noticeable resistance in the process of spinal breathing. There can be several causes.

In the beginning, the most common cause of resistance is the newness of it. We all go through a certain amount of awkwardness as we are learning the practice. The first time we got on a bicycle, did we just ride off smoothly? Of course not. It took some practice, some getting used to. Then, after a while, riding the bicycle became easier. Spinal breathing is like that. There will be degrees of awkwardness. Some will take to it easily, while others may need some time to adjust in the beginning. Keep in mind that it is a simple process, and it does not have to be perfect. All of spinal breathing is a favoring – favoring slow deep breathing, and favoring a pathway inside the spine between root and brow. When we wander off, or feel stuck, we just easily come back to it.

There is another reason for resistance in spinal breathing – obstructions in the nervous system. These are neurobiological restrictions within us that we have carried throughout our life. With spinal breathing, we are coaxing them to relax and release. In the beginning, the resistance from these inner knots can be quite palpable. Some people may find it difficult to pass through a particular area of the inner body with attention and breath traveling up and down inside. The resistance can be found anywhere – the pelvis, solar plexus, heart, throat, or in the head. The resistance can be felt as a blockage that we can't get past, or as some pressure.

What do we do? It is simple. If there is a pressure or a resistance, we just go right by it with our attention and breath. Easily right by it. We never try and force through inner resistance. We just stroke it gently with our attention and breath as we go by. This has a good purifying effect, and will not be uncomfortable. Discomfort comes from forcing against an obstruction. We never do this in spinal breathing. We just whisk on through. What we did not dissolve on the first pass, we will get on the next one, or the next, or the 10,000th pass, maybe years later in our practice. That is how we purify the inner neurobiology. And all the while, we will have the experience of less resistance accompanied by more clarity and fluidity.

With each spinal breathing session, we are journeying deeper within ourselves to realms of greater peace and joy.

Where is the spinal nerve? I can't find it.

Imagine you are a gold miner and you have just staked your claim on a promising piece of land where you believe you will find gold. Maybe you found a fleck or two and are inspired to start digging. Or maybe you bought the claim because you saw the gold others were finding on their claims nearby. Whatever the reason, you start digging, even though you have seen little or no gold. You can imagine the gold being in the earth, so you dig until your imagining becomes the real thing.

Spinal breathing is like that. We imagine the spinal nerve in our traveling up and down with the breath. Will we always be imagining the spinal nerve, or will we actually see it at some point?

As purification advances, our inner experiences will also advance. This is the revealing of the spinal nerve. It is a remarkable discovery we all can make, because we all have a spinal nerve. Every person has one! Our very existence is the proof of it being there. Just as the spinal cord is the main highway of the nervous system, so too is the spinal nerve the main highway of our consciousness expressing on this earth. It is through the spinal nerve that we come to know the full extent of our inner dimensions and the source of all that we are.

But we will not likely see all this on the first day of spinal breathing. Well, maybe a glimpse. Enough to know that there is gold in those hills! Enough for us to be motivated to keep up our twice-daily practice – to keep tracing up and down with our visualization of the spinal nerve that goes from our perineum root to the center of our brow, inside the center of our spine in-between. As we imagine traveling that path easily over and over again, it will reveal itself to us, and a whole lot more – more than we ever imagined.

I was in a huge blissful space. What was it?

It was the spinal nerve. Really, that is what it can be like. It is a paradox. How could such a tiny nerve become so big? It is the essential nature of our neurobiology. Our nervous system is the doorway to vast inner space. More than that – it is the doorway to unimaginable peace, intelligence, energy, ecstatic bliss and divine love. All that inside a tiny little nerve. It is infinity in a bottle, and we are the bottle!

We cannot force our way into this. We can gently coax the purification in our nervous system that will eventually reveal what is within us as a full time experience. This is why we do spinal breathing.

Even in that expanded space, the practice will continue. We just easily favor slow deep breathing while tracing the path between root and brow.

The experience can evolve in many ways according to the course of our inner purification. It is not for us to manage the details of it. Experiences are a by-product of our practice. We always favor our practice over the experiences. We don't try and push the experiences out. We can easily favor our spinal breathing practice with any kind of experience going on, even a glorious expansion inside. This is important.

Everyone has a different purification process, depending on what the matrix of obstructions is within. So the revealing of our inner space can come in many ways. It can come as certain colors, sometimes accompanied by white light. It can be more in the feeling realm, like touching our inner dimensions. It can be with sound, taste or smell. All of our senses operate in inner space.

But none of this is the final destination of spinal breathing. We are going in so we can come back out and enjoy our inner qualities in the outside world of our everyday living. So spinal breathing is a practical technique. It is not something we do to escape. It is something we do to arrive completely in the presence of who and what we are. Then we are in a position to live life to the fullest.

When we come to know that we are infinite inside, then we will see that everything around us in the world is of this same quality – infinite. This we do not have to imagine, for it will become our direct perception. By visualizing the spinal nerve in our spinal breathing practice, we not only discover the spinal nerve, but, ultimately, the nature of everything and everyone we see and interact with in our everyday life. This raises the quality of our life to a new level.

The journey to inner space makes a lot of sense. By going within we will come to know the answer to the question, "What am I doing here?" We are here to discover the truth within ourselves, which is then reflected in everything we see around us.

Enhancing the Effectiveness of Spinal Breathing

By now you may have noticed that there is more to spinal breathing than meets the eye. Make no mistake about it. We are applying one of the world's most sophisticated technologies here. With one simple breathing technique, we are opening our vast inner cosmos, which has profound implications in our outer world. When cultivated correctly, the human nervous system can reveal great wonders and change the quality of our life dramatically. We are the doorway that joins the inner and outer realities of existence, and we can know this by direct experience.

What we have covered so far is the essence of spinal breathing – slow deep breathing while tracing the spinal nerve between root and brow, upward on inhalation and downward on exhalation. This is it, the simplest control lever for utilizing breath combined with attention to transform our presence in the human nervous system into an ongoing cosmic experience. Spinal breathing, followed by deep meditation, will take us surely along the path toward inner peace, creativity, boundless energy and happiness in our daily life.

Now we'd like to consider adding several new features to our spinal breathing that will help improve the effectiveness of the practice. Consider these to be optional, to be taken on or not as you see fit. While basic spinal breathing is quite simple and effective, other things can be done to enhance its influence in the nervous system. That is true of pranayama in general, so it is possible to find a lot of complexity in the many schools of pranayama. Here we will try and keep it simple. At the same time, we will not ignore some means that can be applied to enhance the effectiveness of our practice. We are always open to that, as long as we do not find ourselves running off on tangents that can dilute our practice.

Here we will look at four additional features that can be incorporated into our spinal breathing practice. There is still more that can be added to our spinal breathing routine as we advance, and these methods can be found in the other AYP writings covering mudras, bandhas and related topics. Adding the following four features will be more than enough to bring our spinal breathing practice up to near industrial strength. Don't take these on all at once. Once you are comfortable with what you have learned so far, try one, find stability with it in your daily practice routine, and then add on another, if you are so inclined, and so on. It could be days, weeks or months between additions. Never is okay too. It is up to you. If it ever seems like too much, then just back off and stay at your comfortable level of practice, knowing that with slow deep breathing while tracing the spinal nerve, you have the essentials of the practice well in hand. Everything after that is the icing on the cake.

Full Yogic Breathing

In some schools of pranayama, you don't get to learn how to do any pranayama until you learn how to breathe, yogically that is. That is a little unfair. After all, everyone knows how to breathe. If we did not, we would not be here, would we? So, for the sake of making immediate progress we have jumped right into spinal breathing pranayama, no questions asked. If you can breathe and visualize a bit, you are in. That is almost everyone, yes?

Now that you are in, we can suggest full yogic breathing, so you can get the most out of your spinal breathing pranayama. What is full yogic breathing?

Put simply, it is healthy breathing. Not only that, it is breathing that goes up the body on inhalation, and then back down the body on exhalation, so it fits right in with spinal breathing pranayama. Let's describe it.

Due to the hurried nature of our lives and, sometimes, clothing restrictions, we often tend to be *chest breathers*, meaning that we do most of our breathing in the chest. Full yogic breathing begins lower than that, in the abdomen. Everyone has heard of *belly breathing*, yes? Yogic breathing begins there. When we inhale, we start in the abdomen. This is using the diaphragm to pull down on the lung cavity, expanding it to draw in air. As we do this, the belly goes out – hence the phrase, *belly breathing*. This is natural inhalation, and it is how we used to breathe as babies before we encountered the pressures of the external world.

To continue the full yogic breath, once the diaphragm has reached its comfortable limit in expanding and filling the lungs, we expand the chest cavity as we normally do in chest breathing. We began with the abdomen. Now we expand the chest to bring in more air. Once we have reached a comfortable limit with that, then, finally, we do a slight lift of the collar bones to fill the last small space in the top of our lungs with air. And all of that, going from abdomen, through the chest to the collar bones, is the inhalation stage of a full yogic breath.

Exhalation is a simple reversal of what has just been described. First we let go with the collar bones. Then we let the chest go to expel air. And finally, we let the diaphragm go up, enabling the lungs to move back to their minimum capacity. And then it begins again with the next inhalation.

With some practice, the entire full yogic breath can be done smoothly without effort, with one fluid motion on inhalation and another fluid motion on exhalation. It is easy to make a habit of it in our spinal breathing practice. It enables us to process more air, and this improves the efficiency of spinal breathing overall. Full yogic breathing will become something we do not even think about in spinal breathing, and our attention will be tracing the spinal nerve just as we have discussed already.

As mentioned, full yogic breathing is also healthy breathing and can bring us practical benefits in daily life. Not that we would go around consciously doing it all day long. That would not be very practical. But we do find that, as we develop the habit of full yogic breathing in our spinal breathing, over time, the habit of full yogic breathing will also be showing up automatically in our daily life without even thinking about it. This, in fact, is a fundamental principle in all yoga practice. We expand our inner presence and relaxation in spinal breathing, and, over time, we find more and more of that inner expansion and relaxation in daily life. The same is true of doing deep meditation (more inner silence in life), yoga postures (more flexibility in life) and other yoga practices on a daily basis. It all ends up enhancing our life outside the practices. This is the real benefit of doing yoga practices, and the primary reason for doing them. Using full yogic breathing in spinal breathing pranayama is part of this, and it will effortlessly migrate from our daily practice into our daily life as well, bringing more relaxation and better health along with it.

Opening on Inhalation – Restricting on Exhalation

When we engage in spinal breathing, it is possible to regulate the passage of air through our throat in a way that enhances the process. This is done by opening the throat wider than usual during inhalation, and by restricting it using the epiglottis during exhalation. In doing so, we can achieve better control of the air flow, particularly during exhalation, and enhance the *restraint* aspect of our pranayama. Recall that pranayama means restraint of prana (breath).

As we are inhaling slowly and deeply, while tracing the spinal nerve upward from root to brow with our attention, we can let our throat relax and become larger than usual in the back. This is not an extreme thing – only a favoring of a wide open throat in the back. This produces a beneficial stimulating effect in the area behind the throat area in the upper spine and medulla oblongata (brain stem). It is only done during inhalation.

As we are exhaling slowly, while tracing the spinal nerve downward from brow to root with our attention, we can gently restrict the outward flow of air from our lungs by partially closing the epiglottis, the flap located at the base of our tongue. The epiglottis is used for closing the windpipe when we swallow, and for closing the windpipe when naturally holding our breath. When exhaling in spinal breathing, we close the epiglottis in a way that produces a slight hissing sound deep in our throat, and this is what regulates the exit of air from our lungs. This restriction enables us to extend our exhalation in time (it is okay for exhalation to take longer than inhalation), and also places some positive pressure in the lungs during exhalation, which stimulates the purifying and opening effects of our spinal breathing pranayama.

We do not use this sort of restriction during inhalation for two reasons: First, we want to take advantage of the benefit of the throat opening aspect of practice during inhalation and the stimulation of the brain stem it provides. And, second, restricting the air flow with the epiglottis during inhalation creates negative pressure in the lungs, which is not healthy for the lungs if done over an extended period of time in practices.

So, with these two maneuvers in the throat, which will smooth out to become one process as our practice becomes automatic, we are accomplishing several additional functions during spinal breathing which help in the regulation of the practice and enhance its results significantly.

A Gentle Lifting of the Eyes

In our daily practice, we are doing spinal breathing with our eyes closed, easily tracing the spinal nerve up and down as we breathe slowly and deeply in and out. The spinal nerve, which we are stimulating, is the central highway in the nervous system. By enlivening the spinal nerve with the combination of attention moving up and down, and the restraint of breath, we are stimulating the entire nervous system in a way that is both energizing and relaxing on a very deep level. As we advance in this through our daily practice over time, a gradual awakening will occur which we call *ecstatic conductivity*. This is first noticed as a pleasant sensation that seems instantly connected throughout the body. As it develops, what we find is that this rising experience of ecstatic conductivity is stimulated and regulated from the brain, which does, in fact, comprise the upper end of the spinal nerve. Of particular importance is the region from the point between the eyebrows going back behind it to the center of the brain. This area of the neurobiology in the brain has been called the *third eye*. It is stimulated as part of our normal spinal breathing. To enhance our spinal breathing, some additional stimulation can be provided in this area by developing the habit of a gentle lift of the eyes during spinal breathing. This is not anything extreme or heroic – only a slight lifting of the eyes. As we do this, we can also place a very slight furrowing intention on the center of the brow. Not enough to physically furrow the center of the brow. Only enough to feel some physical intention there. This gentle lifting of the eyes, combined with the slight furrowing intention, places extra stimulation in the area just described as the third eye – the upper end of the spinal nerve.

It is important to note that this is a physical addition to spinal breathing, not a mental addition. As soon as the gentle lifting of the eyes with the slight furrowing becomes habit, we will be giving it no attention at all. It will just be a physical habit, and a slight one at that. Our attention is always for favoring the tracing of the spinal nerve during spinal breathing pranayama. Anything else we may be doing in spinal breathing is only given enough attention to cultivate it to become a physical habit. Then we do not think about it anymore. This goes for our full yogic breathing, opening and restricting in the throat, and the gentle lifting of the eyes. None of these are mental techniques, only a physical habit we are developing to provide particular effects while we are doing spinal breathing. Ultimately, when all of the physical aspects of spinal breathing have become automatic habits, then the only mental procedure we are doing in spinal breathing is the easy tracing of the spinal nerve up and down. This is very important.

In fact, as we advance in our practices, and if we are so inclined, there are additional physical means that can be added to our spinal breathing. Some of these are alluded to later in this book, with detailed instructions available in other AYP books.

If we ever find ourselves in the position of being continually distracted from tracing the spinal nerve up and down during spinal breathing, then we may be trying to add too many elements on at one time. If we are trying to develop full yogic breathing, opening and restricting in the throat, adding the eye lift and other elements into our spinal breathing all at the same time, then it can become difficult to practice effectively. Better to take on each element one at a time letting each become a habit not requiring attention before taking on another. In this way we can gradually build up our spinal breathing practice without putting undue strain on the overall practice.

Cool and Warm Currents

There is a natural tendency in spinal breathing for ascending energy to be cool and descending energy to be warm. When we are able to perceive this and incorporate it into the tracing of the spinal nerve with our attention, it can help us in perceiving the spinal nerve and in more effectively purifying and opening our neurobiology throughout the body.

There is a method we can use for enhancing this process of noticing the cool and warm currents in our spinal breathing.

If we purse our lips and inhale, we can notice the coolness of the air passing through them on the way into our throat and lungs. If we purse our lips and exhale, we can feel the warmness of the air passing out from our lungs through our throat and lips. Now if we do this without pursed lips, we can still notice the coolness and warmness of the air passing into and out of our lungs, yes? We can also notice this coolness and warmness if we close our mouth and breathe through our nose, can't we? Can you feel it now?

This is what we use in spinal breathing. It is a simple transference of sensation (coolness and warmness) felt in the throat and lungs to the path of our attention in spinal breathing – up and down the spinal nerve. It can be part of tracing the breathing up and down the spinal nerve. In addition to taking the breath along with us up and down the spinal nerve, we can also take the sensations of coolness and warmness with us on that journey to inner space. In doing so, we can enhance the effectiveness of our spinal breathing practice.

In time, this becomes a habit, just like the other additional features we have been discussing here. As always, the attention will be traversing the spinal nerve during our spinal breathing. The additional features, if added on prudently, step-by-step, will enhance the effectiveness of our practice.

Always take your time in developing new aspects of practice, whether it be adding on spinal breathing in front of deep meditation, or adding deep meditation after spinal breathing. Always be sure you are stable and comfortable in one practice before attempting to add on another. The same goes for enhancing one of our practices with additional features. If we try and take on too much at once, a simple practice like spinal breathing can quickly become unwieldy. And then we may lose our motivation to practice, which is not doing ourselves a service. So let's always pace the development of our practices to be as smooth and comfortable as possible, knowing that each new element we add will take some adjustment before it becomes an easy habit. If we do this, then there will be no limit to how far we can go with spinal breathing pranayama, or to how deep we can go on our journey to the ecstatic realms of inner space.

The Possibilities

We may begin practicing spinal breathing pranayama for various reasons. Maybe we heard it helps with relaxation. It certainly does. Or perhaps there is a health issue, and pranayama was recommended. Yes, spinal breathing, especially, can do wonders to help balance our inner energies. Often, inner energy imbalances can be the cause of physical health issues. Or we could be coming to spinal breathing pranayama for spiritual reasons, in pursuit of that elusive condition called *enlightenment*.

Whatever our reason has been for starting spinal breathing, it is a good enough reason. It really does not matter why we have begun. The important thing is that we have!

If we commit to a twice-daily practice and give it some time to work, the benefits will be there. The beauty in this is that no matter which of the benefits we have come looking for, we will receive all of the benefits in due course – relaxation, good health and, eventually, enlightenment too.

So the possibilities are very broad – global, we could say. Global within us, and even global around us. Yes, when we take up spinal breathing, we are not only purifying and opening the full range of possibilities within ourselves, we are also opening the possibilities within everyone and everything around us. How can this be?

This was mentioned in the last chapter, how our inner opening can reveal that everything around us is an expression of our own inner consciousness, our own vast inner space. It is an interesting theory, an interesting possibility that we can test for ourselves by engaging daily in spinal breathing pranayama, deep meditation, and other practices. But, the testing of theories aside, there is really only one simple reason for doing this practice – *Freedom*.

We'd all like to be free, which means to be happy in every situation life hands to us, and, above all, to be at peace amidst the fray of life. Once we are in this situation, we are in a position to do the thing that we all inwardly long to be doing – *Giving*.

These two words, *freedom* and *giving*, represent the ultimate possibilities that our spinal breathing practice can deliver. With spinal breathing, we prepare the ground for inner silence to take firm root in our nervous system, and also cultivate the ecstatic inner dimensions within us. These two are the seeds of freedom and giving.

In stillness we find absolute freedom amidst all the circumstances of life. And in the ecstatic flow of our inner realms we find the beginnings of an outward flow from us into our physical environment. This outward flow is a giving, a giving of a very special kind. It is an outpouring of divine love coming through us from within. It is effortless and uplifts everyone and everything around us. As we become free in inner silence and are becoming ecstatically conductive, this process happens all by itself as we go about our ordinary business in daily life.

While life seems to go on in ordinary ways, what is happening in and around us is not so ordinary. We are undergoing the process of human spiritual transformation – the rise of inner silence, ecstatic bliss and outpouring divine love. The consequences of this are extraordinary. Indeed, the world can be transformed for the better by this process, because every heart is lifted up and illuminated by the outward flow of this energy from even only one person.

So the possibilities contained within us are quite profound, and spinal breathing pranayama is one of the primary means for actualizing this great potential for good in ourselves and in the world.

Relaxation? Yes. Good health? Absolutely. Enlightenment? Why not?

Now, let's delve deeper into the practical aspects of managing the process of purification and opening occurring in our nervous system as a result of spinal breathing pranayama.

Chapter 3 – Journey to Inner Space

There is a reason why the word "journey" is used. When we begin the practice of spinal breathing pranayama, we do not instantly arrive in our inner realms. It is a *journey*. We may have tastes of the destination at any time on our journey, but the true arrival will be down the road. There will be a lot of scenery along the way, some of it with the potential for becoming quite distracting, and we will be wise to favor our practice over the scenery. It takes some skill to do this, to travel the road of our purification and opening. In this chapter, we will look in more depth at the kinds of experiences that can come up, and how to regard them to assure our continuing progress.

We will also cover the finer points of spinal breathing, and how to keep our practice steady and stable over the long term. It is long term practice that will bring the greatest results.

Finally, we will look at the flowering of the process – the rise of ecstatic conductivity, the opening of our internal sensory awareness, and the refinement of both of these into a permanent marriage with our unshakable inner silence.

All together, the topics we will cover here can provide a deeper understanding and clarity about what spinal breathing is, how it is done, and the outcomes we can experience in our nervous system as we move ever-closer to our destination.

Managing Our Purification and Opening

As we move along with our daily practice of spinal breathing, many questions come up. These are related to both the mechanics of practice and the resulting experiences. Some of these experiences can be quite exotic. We will deal with these, one at a time, with the aim of bringing clarity to the overall process, so our practice of spinal breathing can continue smoothly and effectively over the months and years. It is through stable long term practice that we come to experience the ultimate results.

The Duration of One Spinal Breathing Cycle

How long does a good spinal breathing cycle take? While it is easy to make it complicated and stressful with all sorts of rules, ratios and the like, it is not complicated at all in the approach we are using here. We do not need a stop watch to practice this easy form of spinal breathing. Neither do we have to struggle to meet any particular time objectives for inhalation, exhalation or overall cycle time. In some approaches to pranayama this is the case. But not here.

The duration of one spinal breathing cycle is the time it takes you to complete one comfortable inhalation and one comfortable exhalation according to the instructions given in the previous chapter. That's it.

The time it takes will be different for each person. It can be different for the same person from day to day, depending on the course of purification occurring in the nervous system. It can even vary in a single spinal breathing session we are doing. Duration is a function of our inner neurobiological processes and our metabolism, which change as the processes of inner purification and opening are occurring.

In spinal breathing we comfortably favor slow deep breathing, whatever that is for us in the moment. That is what determines the duration.

Sometimes our breath will practically stop during spinal breathing. Other times it will go fast. Usually it will be somewhere in-between. All of these scenarios are okay, as long as we are not forcing things one way or the other. It is a natural process.

For those who simply must know what a spinal breathing cycle looks like on the clock, feel free to measure. But please do not set objectives. A short spinal breathing cycle is just as effective as a long one. The body knows what it needs to achieve purification and opening at each and every point in time. In spinal breathing we are providing the body the opportunity to do what it would naturally like to do. As soon as we begin to force the issue we are putting an undue strain on the system which will not necessarily enhance the results.

If pressed on the matter, we can say that a natural spinal breathing cycle duration for most people will fall between fifteen and thirty seconds. It can be less or more, depending on personal factors and the inner dynamics of purification and opening.

Spinal Breathing Session Duration

The duration of our spinal breathing session will be largely determined by what is going on in our nervous system. However, we do not leave the length of our spinal breathing session unregulated. What we do is set a time for practice and stick with that until we have indications in our experiences that we should adjust our time of practice up or down.

When we learn, we begin with five minutes of spinal breathing twice-daily followed by our meditation session. For most people, this will be a good starting time. Once the practice has become smooth and stable, after a few weeks, then we may wish to increase it. Then we can try, say, ten minutes of spinal breathing. With meditation occurring right afterward, this is a healthy amount of practice. More than adequate for most people. Yet, some may like to go higher with the time after the routine has been stable for some time.

The important thing is to find a stable routine – a steady duration of our practice time that we can stick with over the long term. Upward adjustments in our practice time should be made carefully in small steps, and only after our practice has been smooth and stable for at least a few weeks. A few months is better. If we get ahead of ourselves, we will find out soon enough, and that is the time to retreat to a shorter more stable routine of practice. We will discuss that some more in this chapter under "Self-Pacing."

In some schools of pranayama, there is the advice to make pranayama sessions as long as possible – hours in some extreme cases. There is the idea that more is better, as if a certain number of hours of practice in total will equal our enlightenment. If we can do it all by next weekend, so much the better for our evolution. Well, maybe it is so for some teachings, though the evidence is yet to be seen.

Here we take the position that the right session length is a function of each person's inner purification and opening process. There is not a fixed formula for the length of a practice session. It has to be found through each practitioner's experience.

So, five minutes starting out is a guideline, not an absolute. Going to ten minutes for our long term practice is also a guideline. It can be more or less for each person, depending on internal factors. We can only know what it will be for us by gaining some practical experience. Whatever it turns out to be for us, we will be wise to keep our practice duration relatively steady over time. Then we will have a good habit and be in a position to experience ongoing progress with comfort and safety.

Using the Clock Versus Counting Breaths

In the ancient teachings of pranayama, the clock was not used to measure session duration. There were no clocks! Instead, the counting of breaths was used as a measure. And to this day, the counting method is used in many traditional approaches to pranayama, and to other forms of spiritual practice.

In the counting approach, a string of beads is used. In the East this is called a *mala.* In the West it is called a *rosary.* It has other names too. It is a tool for counting and measuring our practice session.

If we are already familiar with the counting approach, we can use it for our spinal breathing pranayama. All we have to do is translate our average cycle time into a count. For example, if our average cycle time is thirty seconds, then five minutes of spinal breathing will be ten cycles of breathing. Ten minutes of spinal breathing would be twenty cycles of breathing, and so on. It can be a little complicated, especially when we consider that our cycle time can vary depending on purification going on inside. So ten cycles of breathing will not necessarily be five minutes of practice. But it can be done that way if there is a strong preference. Those who are already accustomed to using a mala or rosary can certainly use it for spinal breathing too.

For those who are beginning, or looking for an easy approach for measuring session duration, then using the clock will likely be preferred, particularly when we are doing deep meditation right after pranayama, which also is done by the clock.

Add to this the fact that we all have an internal biological clock that can be programmed to be quite accurate, requiring only occasional checking (it's okay to peek), then using the clock to time session duration will be preferred by most. This is, after all, a modern approach to spinal breathing pranayama, with emphasis on ease of use while maintaining maximum effectiveness. The clock is a good tool that aids in achieving these objectives, and is recommended.

Mixing Other Practices with Spinal Breathing

It is easy to add on features to our basic spinal breathing practice. Indeed, it is a great temptation for many practitioners to do so, especially if there has been training in other practices. It is not difficult to find teachings that include spinal breathing loaded down with all sorts of concentration schemes, mantras and more. Often these have a connection with cultural traditions going back hundreds of years.

It has been found that the simplest form of spinal breathing is as, or more, effective than other forms that include many layers of additional practice.

We do add on a few features to the simple form of spinal breathing offered here. We have done so to improve the mechanics of the basic procedure, and none of these additions rely on the division of attention for longer than it takes to cultivate an automatic habit during the practice. This goes for developing full yogic breathing, opening and restricting air flow in the throat, gentle lifting of the eyes, and incorporating the sensation of cool and warm currents into our tracing of the spinal nerve. If we choose to move beyond this initial training in spinal breathing by studying other AYP writings, still more features will be available, but none will be for the purpose of dividing the attention. This is a key point.

In spinal breathing pranayama, it is of vital importance that the attention be free to trace the spinal nerve with minimum distractions and interruptions. This is why we do not try and develop habits for too many additional features of practice at the same time. It is also why we do not "meditate" during spinal breathing.

In yoga, pranayama and meditation are regarded as two separate practices, and in this approach we do not combine them. First we do our spinal breathing pranayama, and then, after that, we do our deep meditation practice. Never the two shall be done at the same time. In this way we take maximum advantage of the simple and effective practice of cultivating the nervous system via the spinal nerve during spinal breathing, and maximum advantage of the simple and effective practice of bringing the mind and nervous system to its deepest levels of stillness through deep meditation. These two practices cannot be done successfully at the same time, and to divide the attention in either of them is to reduce the effectiveness.

Spinal breathing pranayama is the ideal preparation for deep meditation, and deep meditation, done separately afterward, greatly enhances our spinal breathing sessions and overall results over time. Neither practice is a replacement for the other, or a suitable enhancement to be done within the other.

Sometimes when doing spinal breathing, we may find ourselves doing a mantra or some other practice we may have learned at some other time. It is okay if such things come up. We do not favor them. Neither do we try and push them out. We just easily come back to our procedure of spinal breathing, which is slow deep breathing while tracing our spinal nerve between root and brow. This is how we handle diversions that come into our spinal breathing practice. As we will see, diversions can come in many forms, and they are all handled in the same fashion. We always easily favor the procedure of our practice over anything else that comes up during our spinal breathing session.

Alternate Nostril Breathing

A well-known technique that is used for general relaxation and in many systems of yoga is alternate nostril breathing. It consists of closing one nostril with the thumb and breathing slowly out and in, and then switching to close the other nostril with one of the other fingers and breathing out and in again, and so on, alternating back and forth between nostrils.

Though it is certainly possible to use alternate nostril breathing during our spinal breathing practice, it is not recommended. It is redundant with the slow deep breathing we are doing in spinal breathing, and complicates the practice without adding significant results. There are plenty of additional features that can be added to spinal breathing pranayama that produce significant results. Some of these have been covered in this book already, and more are available in the other AYP writings.

If we have been in the habit of using alternate nostril breathing for relaxation, it is okay to continue using it in moderation outside our spinal breathing practice if we feel a strong urge to do so. But be careful not to overdo. If we are practicing more than one kind of pranayama, the effects will be cumulative. That is why it is best for those wishing to undertake spinal breathing to use only the one pranayama technique until the practice routine is well-established and stable. Once that is done, then additional features of practice can be considered one at a time.

Pranayama is a complex field of knowledge, which can bring profound results into our life, if the methods are properly applied. One of the keys in this is keeping it as simple and stable as possible, adding on only those features that will bring us the best results with the least amount of redundancy and complication. It is about efficiency. So, if we have begun our pranayama practice at some time in the past with alternate nostril breathing, this is good. We can leave that behind as we move on to the much more efficient and powerful practice of spinal breathing pranayama.

Spinal Breathing as a Stand-Alone Practice?

In some teachings, pranayama is used as the primary practice, sometimes with an attempt to incorporate elements of meditation into the pranayama. While it may be useful for relaxation, this type of practice does not fulfill the ultimate aim of either pranayama or meditation. Pranayama is for cultivating the neurobiology for a smooth flow of prana, for opening to the inner realms of ecstatic conductivity in the nervous system. Meditation, particularly deep meditation, is for cultivating inner silence in the nervous system – that is, pure bliss consciousness. Pranayama is involved with prana and meditation is involved with consciousness, which is beyond prana. We can be doing one or the other, but not both at the same time. That is why we do our spinal breathing and deep meditation in sequence, and not in parallel.

In some schools, the path is almost exclusively pranayama, sometimes taken to the extreme of many hours of practice per day. In such cases, the results have been seen to be less than optimal. While the nervous system is being opened and made receptive in a pranayama-only approach, there is limited inner silence being introduced due to a lack of deep meditation. This makes the nervous system vulnerable to wayward influences in the mind, emotions and environment, taking such influences deeper into the neurobiology. The result can be an ongoing condition of edginess, irritability, abruptness, inflexibility and a tendency toward anger.

On the other hand, if we use pranayama to purify and open our nervous system, and then cultivate inner silence in deep meditation right after, the long term results will be increasing steadiness, creativity, energy and joy in daily life.

So, while spinal breathing pranayama does not make a good stand-alone practice for the long term, it is a very good complement to incorporate prior to deep meditation. Together, these two practices can serve as the means for promoting safe and effective progress toward unfolding our full potential.

Self-Pacing

Everyone has a different path of purification to travel. This is because we each have come to this place by a different route. The impacts of all past actions and influences on us go back far beyond our recollection, and the obstructions to the flow of energy deep within us are set up accordingly. This is called *karma,* which means action and its embedded consequences. Fortunately, we do not have to remember all that we have done and all that has happened to us. We can gradually unwind all long-lingering internal influences with spinal breathing pranayama and related practices.

The unwinding of all this, and how it happens, is what makes up the particulars of our journey. Purification is often accompanied by some sort of symptoms – often not very noticeable, and sometimes noticeable to the point of distraction. In rare cases the symptoms of purification can be noticeable to the point of near-chaos.

Fortunately, we have a powerful tool to deal with all these various scenarios of purification. We call it *self-pacing*. It is simple, really. Purification and opening can be hastened and stabilized with our daily practices. If purification is happening too fast and uncomfortable symptoms occur, then we slow down our practices until the situation becomes more stable. Once things settle down, then we can inch our practices back up again. This element of self-pacing in our practice routine is very important. Without it, we would all be subject to unnecessary instability on our journey.

Imagine driving a car along a straightaway. The road is smooth and we can travel along at a good pace with safety. Then we come to a mountain and the road begins to wind around, and there are some potholes showing up in the road too. Do we keep going at the same speed we were on the open straight highway? If we do, we might find ourselves flying off the side of the mountain from a sharp curve in the road. It is the same in our practice of spinal breathing pranayama.

Sometimes it will be necessary to slow down while more purification is occurring. Maybe we will cut our time in half, or more, for a few sessions. That is okay. Other times, everything will be smooth, and we can go back to our normal time of practice, with smooth sailing.

Spinal breathing is different from many other yoga practices in that it both stimulates purification in our nervous system and balances our inner energies. This makes self-pacing a little tricky with spinal breathing. If we are experiencing an energy imbalance, a bit more spinal breathing can stabilize the imbalance. This is particularly true with energy finding its way prematurely into certain areas of our neurobiology, like to the crown of the head, or on the left or right side of the spinal nerve. These conditions can be relieved with spinal breathing. Yet, if there is just too much energy running around inside and it is uncomfortable, then backing off on spinal breathing for a few sessions may be the best prescription.

It is a process of getting to know our own inner energy dynamics, and learning how our nervous system responds to different levels of practice. Spinal breathing is a very powerful tool, and we must learn to use it effectively. That will take some testing to determine the cause and effect in our unique energy flow and purification situation.

Self-pacing is also used in making the normal adjustments in our practice times and for adding on the additional features of spinal breathing, as discussed in the last chapter. When we think we are ready for a time increase or a new feature of practice, then we try it. If we over-step and end up with some roughness or too much energy flow, then we step back to our stable platform of practice. Self-pacing.

In this way, we navigate through the varying landscape of our inner purification and opening. Self-pacing is a key tool for this, one that we will always be using for regulating spinal breathing pranayama, and for all of our practices.

Breathing Slowing Down or Stopping
Sometimes we can go deep with our spinal breathing, and breathing can become very slow. Sometimes it can stop for a little while. This is

nothing to worry about. If we are practicing easily and just favoring slow deep breathing, and the breathing slows down or stops, it means our metabolism has gone very low due to the deep relaxation occurring in our nervous system. In that case, the breathing slowing down is not deprivation. We just have less need for oxygen at that time. This is a normal part of spinal breathing that will happen from time to time.

In the ancient lore of pranayama, the cessation of breathing is regarded as a good thing. It is true that a natural slowing or stopping of breathing indicates deep purification, and also that new energies are being awaked within us – more on that later. However, these ancient teachings have often been misinterpreted to mean that forced cessation of breathing beyond normal limits is a good thing. This is not the teaching here, and never will be. Even in other AYP writings where methods of breath retention are discussed, it is never forced beyond our comfortable limit. In any case, this is not what we are doing in spinal breathing pranayama. We go for slow deep breathing while tracing the spinal nerve. If the breathing becomes very slow, or stops, that is fine. Soon we will notice the desire to breathe again, and then we continue our practice just like before. We do not willfully favor the cessation of breathing during our practice. If it happens, it happens. As soon as we notice, we will be wise to easily go back to our normal spinal breathing practice.

Long term progress in spinal breathing is not dependent on breath cessation. It is dependent on a steady routine of slow deep breathing while tracing the spinal nerve.

Sexual Arousal in Spinal Breathing

Sometimes in our spinal breathing session sexual arousal can come. It is a sign of purification and the awakening of our inner energies, and not something to be concerned about. Generally it will pass as purification progresses in our nervous system.

In spinal breathing, we are enlivening and integrating our inner energies from our root to our brow. Obviously, part of this pathway is passing through our sexual neurobiology. And it is also passing through the center of every other part of our nervous system. As the integration of energies within us progresses, our sexual energies will expand upward to become ecstatic. This is usually a gradual development, occurring over the long term as we continue our twice-daily practices. At certain times the symptoms can be noticeable, as in the case of sexual arousal.

The thing to do when sexual arousal occurs is just easily favor our practice of spinal breathing. We may find that the feelings will smooth out higher up in our body. Or they may not. They may be there for the next session, and possibly for several sessions. But eventually they will subside as the resistance unwinds in our neurobiology. Then we may find the feeling expressing ecstatically through our whole body. Or maybe nothing will be going on for a while, and then something later. It depends on the course of our inner purification process, which is unique. The good news is that it is all going somewhere. It is an evolution to higher functioning at work in us, and that is good.

If the sexual arousal becomes so distracting that we find it difficult to practice our spinal breathing, then we can use some self-pacing, as discussed previously. We just back off the time a bit on our practice until the disruptive symptoms of purification settle down. Then we can gradually resume normal practice as appropriate.

For more information on the role of sexuality in the purification and opening of the nervous system, and for means to assist in this natural process, see the AYP writings on *Tantra*.

Energy Flowing in the Body – A New Dynamic

In spinal breathing pranayama we are doing two things at once.

First, we are stimulating the flow of inner energy. This promotes purification and opening in our nervous system, making it a better vehicle for inner silence and pure bliss consciousness, and for the rise of ecstatic conductivity and the radiance of positive energy into our surroundings.

Second, we are coaxing the flow of energy in a way that promotes inner balance – a progressive and stable union of the natural polarities that exist within us. This is necessary so the increasing energy flows do not lead to an energy instability within us. Like any other kind of energy that we utilize in our life, inner energy is a good thing when it is effectively regulated and applied. On the other hand, inner energy can be a problem when it is stimulated and not directed in a productive way.

Both of these functions of spinal breathing, stimulating energy flow and balancing it, are new dynamics that we are bringing into play in our nervous system.

How does pranayama lead to the flow of inner energy? As we restrain breathing in a reasonable and comfortable way as we do in spinal breathing, a slight deficit occurs in our neurobiology. In order to compensate for this slight deficit, the body draws on its vast inner reserve of prana, or life force. This reserve is located in the pelvic region. It is the storehouse of energy normally associated with sexual reproduction. Its broader spiritual function in the nervous system is latent until stimulated in some way. There are a variety of ways this can be accomplished. Pranayama, the gentle restraint of breathing is one of the most effective and reliable ways. This is why, when we are doing spinal breathing, there can sometimes be sexual arousal. But sexual arousal is not a prerequisite for inner energy flow, only an occasional side effect that may occur associated with purification going on in the neurobiology.

The movement of inner energy can be experienced in many ways, in every part of us – physical, emotional and mental. It can also be experienced in the way we perceive our surrounding environment.

As our nervous system becomes purified and opened by the flow of inner energy in a balanced way, our capacity for experience is enhanced. Our sensory machinery becomes greatly refined, and we find ourselves a witness to dynamic inner and outer energy vistas that we could not see before. In this way, all of life within and around us becomes radiant.

Perspiration During Spinal Breathing

Spinal breathing gives rise to whole new dimensions of experience. On the way to this happening, a lot of purification will be occurring in the nervous system, and the symptoms of this are numerous. Inner purification continues throughout the entire process long after the initial inner energy flows from pranayama have become noticeable.

One of the more easily observable symptoms of purification during spinal breathing is perspiration, which can be a direct result of pranayama. This is not perspiration from exertion or exercise. It comes simply from restraint of breath. We may be perfectly comfortable sitting, doing our spinal breathing, and the next thing we know we may be perspiring profusely. It is normal during the early stages of pranayama, and generally will subside as purification progresses. It is not a prerequisite for progress, so if it is not happening, its absence need not be lamented. Everyone is different in this. It is mentioned here so practitioners will know that perspiration is normal if it occurs … and it will pass.

Changes in Digestion

Along the way, we may also notice changes in other tangible functions within our body.

Digestion plays a key role in the process of human spiritual transformation. Spinal breathing pranayama promotes an evolution to a higher form of digestion that involves more than the digestion of food. The combination of food, air absorbed increasingly through the cellular structure of the body during pranayama, and the rise of energy from the pelvic region, all together contribute to the development of this higher form of digestion in our gastrointestinal tract. It can be noticed as additional activity (gurgling) in the digestive system, and as an inner luminosity, an unmistakable glowing sensation arising in the bowels which radiates a refined substance outward through the whole body. As part of this process, the body naturally becomes more porous on the cellular level to the flow of air and the refined essences emanating from the digestive tract and traveling everywhere in our neurobiology.

This remarkable development is a step forward in the rise of an ecstatic radiance coming from within us. The unique functioning associated with this process eventually encompasses the entire body, and will be seen with our inner senses occurring everywhere inside us. In this way we become increasingly radiant from within, and gradually develop an ability to uplift everyone around us with this natural ecstatic radiance. Spinal breathing pranayama plays a key role in this.

Electric-Like Currents and Jolts

As part of the overall process of purification we may sometimes feel electric-like currents inside our body. These can come suddenly and be quite unexpected. They are not common, but it can happen. They generally do not last, and are an indication of energy moving suddenly through obstructions. As the obstructions are dissolved, then the energy flow will smooth out. If currents in the body ever become uncomfortable, then the principle of self-pacing should be applied, and our practice should be reduced in time until the energy becomes smooth again. This goes for any energy excesses we might experience as a result of spinal breathing pranayama or any other practice we may be doing.

Benefit of Yoga Postures and Exercise

Doing some light yoga postures before our spinal breathing can aid in preparing the nervous system for both pranayama and meditation. The logical sequence of practices is postures, pranayama, and meditation – beginning with the body, and going progressively deeper with breathing and mind. If we are doing a comfortable routine of these twice-daily in our practice sessions, then our progress will be enhanced.

If we are not familiar with yoga postures, a class can be taken just about anywhere. Other AYP writings cover postures (also called *asanas*) as well. It takes only five or ten minutes of a well-rounded routine of postures to provide a good foundation of inner flexibility and relaxation in the nervous system. From there, we can go into our spinal breathing and meditation sessions with the opportunity for achieving deeper purification and opening. This is how these categories of practice work together to bring us more quickly along our path.

Some systems involving yoga postures are designed to give us a rigorous physical workout rather than the gentle stretching and relaxation that prepares us for pranayama and meditation. *Power yoga* and rigorous physical exercise is best not done right before our sitting practices. However, a well-conceived program of physical exercise is a good thing to be doing after our sitting practice sessions as a part of our normal daily activities. Exercise at any time other than right before our practice helps stabilize and ground the energies we are cultivating in our spinal breathing pranayama. After our sitting practices, it is good to go out and be active in the world in whatever way we are naturally inclined. This is very beneficial for facilitating a smooth progression of our inner purification.

Automatic Yoga and its Consequences

One of the more noticeable aspects of experience that can result from spinal breathing pranayama is something we call *automatic yoga*.

Automatic yoga is a response in our nervous system that has some recognizable quality that we find somewhere in the broad system of yoga. It is something automatic that happens, as though our nervous system already knows how to do a yoga practice and spontaneously begins doing it. The truth of the matter is that our nervous system already does know all of yoga. The systems of yoga that have been developed over the centuries simply mirror what the human nervous system has taught us about its natural ways of purifying and opening itself. Yoga systems do not define what yoga is. The human nervous system does! We don't even have to call it *yoga*. The same methods have emerged and been given many names around the world. They all have been derived from the human nervous system. The human nervous system is the common denominator in all methods of spiritual practice. The phenomenon of automatic yoga provides some evidence of this.

Automatic yoga comes in many forms. If we begin spinal breathing followed by deep meditation, we may find an increased desire to engage in spiritual studies. Suddenly we will find ourselves reading more books on spiritual matters. We may also notice our conduct becoming more agreeable and kind. Spiritual study and exercising kindness both fall into a category of yoga practice having to do with conduct. Pretty subtle changes, yet noticeable.

The more dramatic and convincing kinds of automatic yoga involve physical movement and postures. The kinds that can come up during or after our spinal breathing practice are automatic suspensions of breath, sudden bellows-like exhalations, or even rapid breathing (panting) that has nothing to do with any external physical activity. Sometimes the head can go down or back. Sometimes it can rotate around as though automatically clearing energy in the neck. The entire torso can lean forward, and, in less-common instances, can lurch, bringing the entire body off the seat. The anus can go into gentle compressions. The eyes can go up. The tip of the tongue can go back on the roof of the mouth. These are all manifestations of automatic yoga. There are many more that can happen. Or there may be none. Automatic yoga is not a prerequisite for progress.

What do we do when a form of automatic yoga occurs during our practice session? It is very simple. We just favor the procedure of the practice we are doing – in this case, spinal breathing pranayama.

So, if we are going along with our spinal breathing and realize that we have stopped breathing without any intention to do so, then we just easily pick up where we left off and continue with our slow deep breathing as we trace the spinal nerve. If we don't remember where we were when we went off into the automatic yoga, then we just start over at the root with a new inhalation, and go from there.

The same is true if we find ourselves in rapid breathing, or in some other form of movement. We just ease back to the procedure when we realize we have gone off into something else.

The question may arise, "If automatic yoga is *automatic*, why don't we let go of our structured routine and just go with the automatic yoga?"

There are several reasons why we don't do this. First, while automatic yoga is impressive (a confirmation!) it is not very systematic. While an automatic breath suspension may happen, it does not know what is supposed to happen next to facilitate the effective integration of its effects. Such integration is essential if we are to stay on a stable path of purification and opening. Automatic yoga is not capable of keeping us on a regular routine of practice either. It is the raw expression of our spiritual energies. It is up to us to utilize the tendencies within us in a systematic way to achieve the desired results. Some of the automatic yogas we may experience are found in specific practices we can learn to use in a systematic way in other AYP writings.

Second, if automatic yoga is left to its own devices, it can lead us into excesses that will be difficult to assimilate. The truth is that automatic yoga, while a very significant phenomenon, does not care about the well-being of our body, or our emotional and mental state. It is the raw force of nature attempting to purify and open us all at once. It will try and do it all today if we will allow it. But that is not possible, so, in that sense, automatic yoga is not practical in the moment. It is our innate spiritual energy expressing itself.

Intense spiritual desire is also like that, having great power to transform us. It too is an automatic yoga that arises from our practice. If taken to extremes, spiritual desire can lead to irrational acts that can harm us. So spiritual desire must be tempered and utilized within the realm of what is practical. Spiritual desire (in some form) has brought us to spinal breathing, and our practice will increase our spiritual desire further.

This cautionary advice about automatic yoga does not mean we do not take a chance now and then. Sometimes we will let it go, let the breath automatically suspend, or whatever. In a sense, all practices are automatic. We do them because we feel we must in order to grow. In doing so we will inevitably run into some excess energy flows from time to time, and then we will be wise to self-pace our practices accordingly. It is all for the good – for our purification and opening, and for a higher quality of life all the way around.

Up to this point, we have looked at the practical aspects of establishing and stabilizing our spinal breathing practice, and managing it in relation to some of the symptoms of purification that we may encounter as we travel along our path. It is necessary for us to develop some skills in order to navigate successfully through the many experiences that can come up.

Now we will go deeper into the more refined aspects of spinal breathing and its effects, looking at several kinds of energy experiences and visions that can occur on the way to inner space. With these kinds of experiences, it is also necessary to exercise some skill in our practice so we will be able to continue making good progress without becoming sidetracked from our path.

Energy Experiences and Visions

So far, we have been discussing the procedure of spinal breathing pranayama and the physical and initial internal energy-related experiences that can come up. We know now that these experiences are related to purification and opening in our nervous system, and that we easily favor our practice over the various experiences that may come up.

Now we will go deeper into the kinds of experiences that can occur during and after spinal breathing pranayama, and see how they relate to our practice. Interestingly, what we will be covering now is only an extension of what we have been discussing already. As our practice advances, and as we see openings occurring along the way, our physical and initial energy experiences will become more refined in their nature and content. It is a crossing over into the realm of *inner space*, where we speak of our experiences less as being perceptible manifestations of energy within us, and more as being *visions*. It is the same purification and opening, going deeper and taking our experiences deeper also. How do we treat these so-called visions when they come up during our spinal breathing practice? In the same way that we treat physical and energy experiences – when we find our attention off into a vision, we just easily come back to our spinal breathing practice.

So we can develop more clarity about what is happening within us as a result of spinal breathing pranayama, let's now look at the phenomena of refined energy experiences and visions from several angles.

Relationship of Energy, Senses, Heart and Mind

First of all, in order to have a vision of any kind, we have to be sensing something, perceiving something. Our sensory machinery has to be somehow engaged. If our experience is refining, it stands to reason that not only are we becoming refined within in a material way, but so too is our ability to perceive what is happening through our senses being refined. It is an integrated process.

All five senses continue to operate as we go inward. As the nervous system becomes more purified and opens in inward ways, we can perceive that the flow of pranic energy within us becomes more refined. It is through the simultaneous refinement of our sensory perception that we can bear witness to the process. If we could not sense it, would it be a happening? Not as far as we could tell.

It is like the old riddle, "If a tree falls in the forest and no one is there to hear it, does it make a sound?" This points to the intimate connection between the observer and the observed. Even if the event did happen, who would know if it were not perceived in some way, either during or after the fact?

In the case of human spiritual transformation, the experience of it is both during and after, and that is what makes practices like spinal breathing so worthwhile – we can perceive our progress and also look ahead to envision a destination. Indeed, we can reach the destination! More on that later.

The machinery of our senses is rooted in stillness, in consciousness. So is all of material existence, including our functioning nervous system through which we experience our inner and outer worlds. If we have been engaging in deep meditation, we know that the mind has its root in stillness also. We have called this stillness *pure bliss consciousness*, or our *being*. The feelings in our heart originate in stillness, as well. Our deepest feelings are in stillness. So we can say that whether we are talking about material existence, sensory perception, feeling, or thinking, all of these are rooted in stillness. In stillness, all of these things are one, and they are intertwined at every level coming outward from stillness into manifestation.

As we practice spinal breathing pranayama and enliven the flow of the life force within us, inner energy will begin to flow. As it does, our inner sensory machinery will deliver the perception and the experience, because the senses are refining at the same time. Similarly, our heart and mind will be enlivened at more refined levels. These components always open together because they are the connected sides of a multi-sided coin. So, as energy begins to flow within us as a result of our spinal breathing practice, our senses, thinking and feeling are all part of this flow, thus endowing us with the various experiences associated with purification and opening, and, ultimately, with enlightenment.

The question may come up, "Is the change in sensory perception all that is happening? Are we just seeing more of our current inner energy, or is there more involved?"

Because increases in inner energy flow are often accompanied by additional symptoms that can be physical, mental or emotional, it is clear that much more than a refinement in sensory perception is occurring. Every aspect of our nature is affected, leading us to progressively refined levels of neurobiological functioning. It is all connected...

Changing Character of the Spinal Nerve

When we begin spinal breathing pranayama practice, we imagine a tiny nerve going from our perineum to the center of our brow, and we trace that up and down with our attention as we breathe slowly and deeply in and out. If we have had some prior experience with our inner energies, then we may find right away that the spinal nerve is a real thing within us. Then we find that we can trace something perceptible instead of imagining the path. Either way, spinal breathing is the same process.

Going from imagining the spinal nerve to sensing it directly in some way (seeing, feeling, hearing, etc.) is a change, not only in our perception, but also in the character of the spinal nerve itself. As mentioned above, the purification and opening going on within our nervous system and the refinement of our sensory perception go together. This progression, this change in the character of the spinal nerve, will go a very long way as we continue with our daily practice over months and years.

There is no precise scenario for how the spinal nerve will change. It depends largely on the condition of our nervous system when we begin our spinal breathing practice. The central nerve in our spine is connected with every other nerve in our body, and even reaches beyond our body energetically. So the purification we are talking about here is very broad, beginning with the tiny nerve in us. And so too does our experience of the spinal nerve become very broad as we continue with our practice over the long term.

If we start at the very beginning with imagining the spinal nerve, we can construct a general scenario for the changes that can occur. The first thing we may notice is a thread-like energy where we have been tracing up and down with our visualization. It can be warm or cool, corresponding to the cool and warm currents we have been promoting with that particular feature of our practice. It can be hot and cold at the same time, like mint. It can take on a silver color and develop a certain intensity about it. We might feel it coming right out of our loins, which gives it a pleasurable sexual coloring. But not entirely sexual. It is something else. Something going up through our center and away from our genitals. Maybe we will feel it going all the way up into our head and out through our center brow as we are doing our spinal breathing. There can be some pressure associated with it at the brow or elsewhere in the head.

We already know that if experiences like this or any others come up, we just easily favor our spinal breathing practice. If there is pressure that becomes uncomfortable, we self-pace our practice accordingly until the pressure subsides. Spinal breathing is not a heroic practice. It is a smart practice.

So maybe a thread-like experience like that will be the first experience we have beyond imagining the spinal nerve. Or maybe it will be something more. Either way, we will know that we are making progress. But it is only a beginning, so we just carry on with our practice…

Once we have a perceptible thread of energy occurring in our spinal breathing, it can only expand. And it does, over time. We can observe this as a thickening of the energy corresponding to our spinal nerve. It can become quite large. As it does, it can become dynamic – moving, swirling and changing color as we observe it up and down. We can do this from the outside, and also from the inside. In fact, our spinal breathing does not change at all through all of this. We still remain at the center of the spinal nerve going easily up and down, no matter how big the swirling currents may become. The procedure of spinal breathing is a great stabilizer in all of this, keeping our inner energies in balance, even as they are increasing in their scope and intensity.

Keep in mind that the drama we might see happening with our inner energies is part of the process of purification going on within us. As our nervous system becomes more pure, the drama will become less, even as the energies are becoming greater and expanding further and further out from the center like a giant spiritual cyclone. And still we will be sitting there quietly during our daily practice, easily doing our spinal breathing just the way we have always done it. Life will go on the way it did before, except we will be much more engaged from within – more alert, more balanced, more creative, and more able to give to those around us than we could before, because we will have so much more to give.

Our actual experience can leapfrog to any level of the scenario just described. It can also go instantly beyond the raw energy experiences to direct experiences of inner space, which we will be getting into next.

The spinal nerve will change in its character as we progress with spinal breathing. It is a normal part of our inner development. As long as we continue to regulate our practice so as to be smooth and stable, then the entire process can be conducted quite naturally. If we find ourselves running off on a tangent, becoming infatuated with our inner experiences, then it is time to easily come back to our simple spinal breathing practice. It is the practice that will carry us forward, not the experience. Let's never forget that.

The Heart Space

While there can certainly be a lot of dynamic energy moving as our nervous system purifies and opens, we will also find profound stillness within it. At times during our spinal breathing, or in our deep meditation that follows, we can find ourselves in a vast empty space. It can be dark, or full of light. We may see nothing in particular, yet know we are in a seemingly infinite space with no boundaries. We may hear sounds, water running, crickets, a bell chiming. We may feel lovingly touched in this space, in ways that make us melt into tears. There can be sweet smells and wonderful tastes. Whatever the experience may be in there, if the space seems unbounded, it will be the heart space.

If we find ourselves in this experience during our spinal breathing practice, we can acknowledge it and then ease back to our practice. It is the practice that has opened us to our inner space, the glorious realms of our heart, and it is our practice that will further that experience in ways that we can scarcely imagine. Our journey to inner space is a long one and it is carried forward by our daily practices. The gorgeous scenery we encounter along the way is only that – scenery. We can enjoy it for a while. If we want to travel further, then we know it is our twice-daily spinal breathing that will carry us forward.

Opening of the Third Eye

We have all heard of the *third eye*. What is it, and what does it do?

From our point of view as knowledgeable practitioners of spinal breathing pranayama, we know that the third eye is nothing more than the upper end of our spinal nerve. And it is being purified and opened in a systematic way along with all the rest of our neurobiology. So there is no extra effort required to be opening the third eye. With spinal breathing pranayama, we are doing it!

Energetically, the third eye can be viewed as the entire spinal nerve. But more commonly, we view it as encompassing the area from the medulla oblongata (brain stem) to the center of the brow. Once the third eye becomes enlivened as part of the energy dynamics of the awakening spinal nerve, it is indeed intimately connected with every part of the spinal nerve from root to brow, and the entire nervous system via that central connection. We call this the rise of *ecstatic conductivity*. It is by this ecstatic connection through the purified spinal nerve that the third eye becomes the master controller of the internal energy aspect of our spiritual evolution. This is not something anyone has to take on faith. It is a palpable experience that comes up as the spinal nerve purifies and opens and the energy flow naturally evolves. Then the ecstatic connection between the third eye and root can be felt clearly and permanently. It is a milestone in our spiritual evolution.

Is the third eye an all-seeing eye? Not in the way we think about seeing. It is has an all-seeing quality that evolves as we come to perceive more and more of our inner dimensions. The inner journey depends on the rise of ecstatic conductivity and the third eye is at the center of that. The third eye is also at the center of rising intuition – which is another kind of seeing. With the spinal nerve becoming increasingly purified and opened, our ability to see the truth of life before us is enhanced dramatically. This is not only in our general perception of things as they are, but also in knowing better the right course of action to take in any given situation. The third eye sees in this way. It is the channel to great wisdom in us, connecting with the deepest levels of mind, heart and the cosmos within and around us. This is the kind of seeing the third eye does.

As the upper part of our spinal nerve purifies and opens we can have many symptoms in the head, including visions, humming sounds (*OM*) and other sensations. In some systems, these intermittent symptoms of purification and opening are used for practice, but not in our approach here.

As long as we are doing our daily spinal breathing practice we will steadily be opening the spinal nerve, and the third eye along with it. Let's not get too caught up in the experiences that we may have in the third eye area, no matter how profound they may seem. Focusing on experiences we may have in the third eye region is not the best means for opening it up, and we will do well to continue with our spinal breathing practice just as we have been before. Then everything will evolve naturally and we will have all the benefits of an opened third eye.

The Tunnel and Star

There is an experience that practitioners of spinal breathing pranayama may encounter. It can happen just about anywhere along the way, or not at all until much later. It is not necessarily a measure of progress, but more of a confirmation. One of many that we can encounter as our practice advances.

Sometimes during spinal breathing a circular vision can appear. It can be very hazy. It can be dark in color, or just about any color of the rainbow. Dark blue or violet is common. The vision can also be two concentric circles with a light outer one and a dark inner one. The vision can be as dramatic as a rainbow of concentric circles going from red on the outside through orange, yellow, green and blue to deep violet in the center, or any partial view of these. There can be flashes of white light in these concentric circles, or a single blazing white star or white point of light in the center of the circular vision. What is all this?

Well, it is simply the view looking up and out through the tunnel of the spinal nerve. The colors are of decreasing density going from the root to the brow, toward the center, and the white light is the view out through the third eye. Is there something out there, a permanent destination we need to go to? No, not now. Perhaps when we reach the end of our life and leave our body, we may experience traveling through a tunnel like this, and into the light. It has certainly been well-documented in studies of those who have had near-death experiences. But that is not what we are doing with spinal breathing pranayama. We are not leaving. We are arriving. We are doing the practice to live a better life here and now on this earth. We are doing it to purify and open our spinal nerve so more of our divine qualities can flow into this life. So we are bringing the light in here, not going out into it to leave this place.

Along these lines, during spinal breathing, if we are inclined to extend the tracing of our spinal nerve outward through the center of our brow and toward a distant point slightly above our brow, slightly above the horizon, then this can be helpful in our practice.

Our spinal nerve does extend that far, and the vision of the tunnel and star is an indication of this. So we can use this knowledge in a practical way. It is an option, not a requirement. If we prefer to keep our tracing of the spinal nerve between the root and brow, this is fine. It is more than enough, and will take care of the entire process of purification and opening from the standpoint of pranayama practice.

What we do not do in this approach is get all involved in the vision itself, if it is occurring. We keep our spinal breathing practice straight-forward and simple – an easy tracing of the nerve. We do not add the elaborate features and dimensions of whatever vision we may be having, as these will change from day to day, or may not be occurring at all. Whatever we see or do not see is fine. The vision is not the practice. The practice is very simple and will produce the necessary results. If we begin adding more visualization to it beyond the simple tracing up and down, the effectiveness of the practice can be reduced.

In some teaching approaches, great importance is placed on having a particular vision, and so much time and effort are invested in having that vision. We do not do that here. As long as we are easily favoring the procedure of our practice, it does not matter if visions or energy experiences are there or not. This is because visions do not produce spiritual progress. The practice of spinal breathing is what produces the results. Let's always keep that in mind whenever we feel tempted to chase after the *sirens of experience*. Just easily come back to the simple procedure of spinal breathing, and all will be progressing fine.

Lower and Higher Beings

There is life in inner space, and we will no doubt encounter it sooner or later. The good news is that it will only be part of the scenery we encounter as we travel along our path. And, by now, we know how to handle scenery, yes? Whatever comes up, we just easily favor the practice we are doing. If visions and inner experiences come up during our daily activities, we just carry on with whatever we are doing. The only way we can become distracted by the happenings in inner space is if we give ourselves to the energy experiences and visions that may appear. It is like taking any other trip. We can just keep driving, or we can stop at every exit and turn-off. It is the choice we make that will determine our progress toward our destination.

Before we began spinal breathing pranayama, maybe we had some experiences with inner beings, most likely ordinary souls like us who are hanging around for whatever reason. It is pretty common. Lots of people have experienced it in one way or another. What will be the effect of spinal breathing pranayama on the tendency to have this kind of experience? It will tend to make it less, mainly because we are making a huge sweep through inner space each time we trace the spinal nerve up and back down during our slow deep breathing. So, localized inner events will fade into the much bigger landscape of our cosmic interior. All that has been described up until now is in the direction of expanding us far beyond the limited spiritual experiences that define the world of psychic phenomena and mediumship. We are leaving all of that behind the minute we sit with spinal breathing pranayama for the first time. This does not mean we will not see anything in the realms of lower beings. But we will certainly not be bound to such things, and can easily choose to let them go in favor of our practice that will purify and open us to a much greater reality within us.

Higher beings are another story. The longer we are practicing spinal breathing, especially if followed by deep meditation, the more we will be in contact with higher beings. What does this mean?

It is not usually in the way we think about being with others, sitting at the kitchen table with the founder and savior of our particular religion. Theoretically, it could happen that way, but it is not likely. Usually, it is much more subtle and much more powerful, and very much within us. Higher beings are *within* us.

Where?

Well, everywhere, but especially in our heart and up through our third eye.

Should we be trying to contact them in these places?

We are already doing it with our spinal breathing. If we are doing our practice with devotion, a huge amount of contact with higher beings will be occurring.

How will we know? By the many blessings that are coming our way.

Do we have to believe in this to receive the results?

Absolutely not. It is a mechanical process of purifying and opening our nervous system. As it opens, whatever is within us becomes available. No matter how we view it, the results will speak for themselves, and we can interpret them however we wish.

The fact is, as we progress with spinal breathing we experience the kinds of things that have been discussed already. We become more centered, more intuitive, more creative, more energetic and more inclined to do good in the world. Something flows through us more and more and out into our daily life, and it is good.

So, there is no need to wait for our savior to ride up in a golden chariot to save us from a life that we are not enjoying. We can practice spinal breathing pranayama and save ourselves, and our savior will be smiling more and more each day from within us. Whatever our religious beliefs may be, as long as we are attuned to revealing the truth, they will fit naturally, because we are getting in touch with that within us which is sacred, and leaving the darkness and our limited views of life far behind. It is a new dawn!

Chakras and Kundalini

In addition to the spinal nerve, there is quite a lot of energy circuitry within us. There are many thousands of nerves that can be identified physically, and experienced directly in our inner realms as purification and opening occurs within us as a result of our daily practice of spinal breathing. Our neurobiology has certain zones, plexuses and regions that have been identified in traditional yoga as *chakras*. These are the energy centers that receive so much attention in the various traditions. Chakra means, "wheel." Chakras may be experienced as whirling wheels of energy located at various locations in the body, and are connected by the spinal nerve. There are seven primary chakra locations – root/perineum, internal sexual neurobiology, naval/solar plexus, heart, throat, third eye (brow to brain stem), and the crown of the head.

Chakras are not part of the actual practice of spinal breathing pranayama in the style we are presenting here. We do not focus on them as part of our practice. They do play a role in the inner mechanics of what results from the simple method of spinal breathing we are using, in the same way that the engine and transmission in a car play a role when we are operating the vehicle with the simple controls – the steering wheel, gas pedal and brake pedal. When we step on the gas pedal, the car moves. When we turn the steering wheel, the car turns. When we step on the brake, the car slows down and stops. We do not have to be thinking about the complex operations of the engine, transmission and all the other machinery that is under the hood of the car while we are doing these things. Thank goodness! We could not drive the car very easily if we had to attend to every single detail going on under the hood while we are driving.

It is like that with spinal breathing and chakras. The chakras are there and are part of the internal operations. But we do not have to manage the details of those inner operations. If we are easily engaged in our spinal breathing practice of slow deep breathing and tracing the spinal nerve up and down with our attention, then all the rest will happen automatically, as we have been discussing already in this book. If we find ourselves drawn to some energy experience during our spinal breathing practices, it may be related to activities going on in one or more of our energy centers, or chakras. What we do is always the same in situations when we are having an experience. We just easily go back to our practice of spinal breathing. It is very simple. So, whatever is going on inside, we just favor the procedure. There is no need to get all wrapped up in considering this or that energy experience, or this or that chakra. It is all under the hood. We just stay with the main controls in our spinal breathing, and we will be moving swiftly along the road on our way home.

The reality of inner energy flow in the human nervous system can be verified by anyone who takes up spinal breathing pranayama and other practices that we discuss in the AYP writings. The natural process of awakening our inner energies through the purification and opening of our neurobiology has been described in mythological terms over the centuries in many cultures around the world. Yoga has an elaborate mythology describing the natural processes that occur in every human being as practices are undertaken and spiritual awakening occurs. Christianity has a mythology too. All religions and cultures do, because wherever there are people discovering their spirituality, the experiences come up and are described in some way that is suitable to the culture and religious beliefs. But it is the same experience, you know, determined by the inner functioning of the human nervous system.

At the heart of yoga mythology is something called *kundalini*. Kundalini means, "coiled serpent." This refers to the vast storehouse of prana (life force) residing in the pelvic region of everyone. It is our sexual energy. Until it is awakened and brought into active manifestation in the nervous system, it is latent potential, or coiled. The serpent aspect depicts the ability of this latent potential energy to become active and move through us along a narrow path – through the spinal nerve. So this is what kundalini is in the simplest terms. It is the gentle awakening of energy within us as a result of spinal breathing pranayama. As purification and opening advances within us, it is regulated smoothly and safely by our spinal breathing. Then we find ourselves having increasing access to our inner realms, as previously discussed. It is important to note that a mythology that has been constructed in ancient times to describe a natural phenomenon within us does not determine the phenomenon itself. The natural tendencies for growth contained within each of us determine what will happen. We have the means to stimulate our natural tendencies with spinal breathing to awaken our own inner nature. When we do, what we see will be our own, and we will interpret it on our own ground within the context of our experience and cultural or religious background.

Spinal breathing pranayama will work within any cultural or religious framework, or with no cultural or religious framework at all. It is a neurobiological transformation we are engaged in which opens us to our innate potential. How we relate to our inner opening and journey to inner space is our own business.

So, this discussion on chakras and kundalini is only to provide some basic understanding about these concepts, which we all will hear about sooner or later as we delve into the methods of yoga. The inner mechanics and the classifying of them have little bearing on the actual conduct of our practice, or on how we ultimately choose to interpret our experiences. If anything, we'd like to downplay the tendency many of us have to dwell on this or that mythology, and bring our attention to what really matters the most – our own inner purification and opening that can be easily cultivated via twice-daily practice of spinal breathing pranayama.

Avoiding a Premature Crown Opening

The spinal nerve is a pathway that we are purifying and opening between our root and brow. It is a specific route that we are opening for specific reasons. First, the spinal nerve is the main highway of the body's vast and complex system of energy pathways. By purifying and opening this specific root-to-brow pathway, we are assured of purifying and opening the entire nervous system in a progressive, smooth and safe way. There are other ways to do it that may be considered to be progressive, but may not be regarded as smooth and safe.

One way that leads many into great difficulty is the so-called *crown opening* route. Perhaps the question has come to mind already, "Why don't we do our spinal breathing between root and crown instead of root and brow?" The answer is simple: Purifying the spinal nerve between root and crown in spinal breathing has the potential to produce huge and unstable energy flows in the nervous system. In fact, any sort of crown practice that is done before sufficient prerequisite purification has been achieved can lead to large and unstable inner energy flows.

So, the caution here is, avoid a premature crown opening.

This will not be a concern if twice-daily root-to-brow spinal breathing pranayama is utilized. The involvement of the third eye as a natural part of our spinal breathing practice, combined with self-pacing, ensures that the purification and opening in the head will be smooth and stable. The third eye has this stabilizing quality, and that is the primary reason why our spinal breathing traces the route in the head the way that it does – for a smooth, stable opening, and good control of the overall process of energy awakening in the whole body. The ancient Sanskrit word for the third eye is *ajna*, which means "command." That says it all, doesn't it?

Interestingly, by engaging in our daily root-to-brow spinal breathing over time, the crown is opened in a natural way in the correct sequence with the rest of our body's neurobiology. When the crown opening occurs in this way, as a by-product of overall spinal nerve awakening via root-to-brow spinal breathing, then the risk of crown-related energy problems is greatly reduced.

Root-to-brow spinal breathing is such an effective energy balancing practice that, in cases where an unruly premature crown opening has occurred previously, root-to-brow spinal breathing practice can go a long way toward stabilizing and correcting the problem. So, not only is spinal breathing pranayama an excellent tool for advancing our inner purification and opening, it can also be a remedy, at least in part, for energy problems that can occur when inner openings are out of balance.

We have looked at many aspects of spinal breathing pranayama, and the kinds of experiences that can occur over time as a result of our twice-daily practice. The focus has been on the practical application of this important breathing technique, and managing our practice in a way that enables us to navigate through the ever-expanding landscape of our inner realms. No matter what we may notice happening along the way, our continued progress will always depend on easily favoring the procedure of our practice over the experiences that come up during our sittings. If we are having experiences of inner space while we are engaged in our daily activity, well, we can just enjoy them. Our rising inner experiences will not be a barrier to us accomplishing our duties during the day. As a matter of fact, our inner energy flow can greatly enrich our functioning in daily life, filling everything we do with peace, creativity, energy, love and joy.

Now let's take a look at ecstasy, a primary quality we are developing within ourselves with our spinal breathing practice. We will also discuss how ecstasy combines with inner silence, a primary quality we develop in deep meditation. These two together, ecstasy and inner silence, are the lynch-pins of enlightenment.

The Evolution of Ecstatic Conductivity

The human nervous system has a capacity for ecstatic pleasure that far exceeds what most of us can imagine. We don't have to be shy to say this, or hesitant to systematically go about cultivating it as part of our normal everyday life. Joy and happiness are our birthright, and the experience of ecstasy is an important part of this. If it is approached in the right way, it will not be hedonistic – for pleasure only. Ecstasy can be refined in a way that is in direct support of our spiritual progress. In fact, ecstasy is an essential part of our spiritual progress toward higher stages of development. Without it, we will not have the whole thing. Enlightenment is not possible without ecstasy!

There have been references in our discussion so far to *ecstatic conductivity* and *ecstatic radiance*. The first leads to the second, and both are cultivated in spinal breathing pranayama over the long term. It is a natural evolution, which we are able to nudge steadily forward with our practice, much the way we enable a plant to grow strong and mature with prudent fertilization and watering.

With spinal breathing we are enabling our inner energies to come to life and express in a higher way within us. It is a gradual process. It begins as we awaken the relationship between our spinal nerve and the vast storehouse of sexual energy in the pelvic region. As we do our spinal breathing, the spinal nerve is purified and opened and our latent sexual energy is stirred ever-so-gently to awaken and find its relationship with the spinal nerve and our higher neurobiology. The symptoms of this unfolding event can vary. Earlier, it was described as a pleasant sensation rising in the spinal nerve – a thread-like sensation of ecstatic pleasure rising from the pelvic region and going up. The sensation can traverse the entire spinal nerve from root to brow instantly. It is less of a gradual traveling upward, and more of an instant lighting up of the thread-like spinal nerve with luminous pleasure. Then we can stimulate that by moving our eyes gently upward and furrowing our center brow in an inward way – no big external physical movement. We can stimulate the feeling from there, from the region of the third eye. It is a connection. Our spinal nerve is *conducting* the ecstatic energy like an electric current. The third eye becomes like a switch and a volume control that can be used to increase or decrease the intensity of the ecstatic current. This is the beginning of ecstatic conductivity.

From this beginning, the ecstatic current will work its way out into the many thousands of nerves throughout our body. We will feel it in our arms and hands, and in our legs and feet. We will feel it in our sexual organs (sometimes arousing), in our belly, in our heart, our throat and mouth, and in our head, including at our crown. It is okay to feel it at the crown – it is a natural opening, not one we are pushing to excess to be out of balance with our whole-body opening. Ecstatic conductivity, naturally centered in the spinal nerve between root and brow will provide for this balanced opening in every nerve of the body. And it happens simultaneously everywhere in us due to the electric current-like nature of our ecstatic energy. But it is not full purification and opening on the first day. Not even in the first year will this process likely be complete. As we continue with our spinal breathing, the process will continue over a long time, and we will see it evolve through a seeming never-ending expansion.

The thread-like ecstatic spinal nerve expands to become like a rope, then like a column, and finally a vast field of energy that reaches far beyond our body.

Even in thread-like mode, our ecstatic conductivity has a radiant quality about it. Like when an electric current travels through a wire, a field is generated whose influence can be felt beyond the wire. In science, it is called *electromagnetism*. It is the principle upon which all electrical machinery operates – currents producing magnetic fields and vice versa. A similar principle exists with the movement of ecstatic energy within our nervous system. As the inner flow increases, the radiation of ecstatic energy increases also. The increasing ecstatic conductivity within us produces radiance. We call this *ecstatic radiance*.

Of course, the purification and opening in each of us is different according to the matrix of inner obstructions. But the underlying vehicle of our nervous system is the same, and as the obstructions are gradually dissolved, the divinely ecstatic experience that shines through from within is one we share in common with all human beings.

How we arrive at that can vary. Spinal breathing pranayama is an equalizer in that it balances the ascending and descending energies within us, greatly reducing the tendency some may have for energy lurches, heat, cold, emotions, visions and other symptoms that can come up as a byproduct of our inner purification.

While the evolution of ecstatic conductivity expands and the flow of energy greatly increases, there will also be a reduction of the symptoms of purification as time goes on. Why is this?

It is because, as our spinal nerve and all the rest of our neurobiology becomes purified, there will be less resistance to the flow of inner energy. Obstructions in our nervous system create *friction* as energy passes through. As the obstructions dissolve, the friction becomes less, and the flow becomes very smooth. As the evolution of our ecstatic conductivity continues in this direction, we are able to conduct much larger flows of inner energy without the resistance we experienced before. In fact, in the end, we will have vast amounts of divine energy flowing through us, and may not even notice. But others will, because the greatly increased inner energy flows will produce greatly increased ecstatic radiance in all directions around us. In this way, our energy influences others without us having to do anything other than attend to our own inner evolution. Of course, we will be doing more than that, because with the increasing ecstatic radiance comes a greatly increased outflow of love and compassion. And so, we will be more inclined to act for the benefit of others. Ecstatic radiance has both an invisible energy component and a physical component embodied in our actions.

So ecstatic conductivity yields ecstatic radiance, and ecstatic radiance yields ecstatic action for the benefit of all. It is an irresistible radiation of divine love coming from within us. This is the fruit of spinal breathing pranayama.

In order for this evolutionary process to progress something more is needed – inner silence. The full flowering of enlightenment involves a special dynamic occurring deep within our inner realms. It is the marriage of two aspects of our nature, which constitutes an advanced evolutionary stage in our nervous system, leading to the completion of the process of human spiritual transformation. It is the marriage of our dynamic ecstatic conductivity with our immovable inner silence – and these two become One.

Chapter 4 – The Cosmic You

Where is inner space? Where is the legendary kingdom of heaven where "all is added" to us? The answer seems obvious enough, doesn't it? It is within us!

Yes, this is the direction we must take. Yet, it seems opposed to so much of what we are doing in the world – where we are engaged in our daily commitments, making a living, raising a family, seeking some peace and fulfillment in our life, and all that. Like so many things having to do with spiritual matters, there is a paradox. Things are not always what they seem. By going inward we can have the greatest effect on our external life, a far greater impact than anything we can do in our outer life.

So we go within with our spinal breathing and our meditation, and, surprisingly, things on the outside get better – more peace, more energy, more creativity, more happiness...

Then, somewhere along the way, we make an astounding discovery. We find that the inner space and kingdom of heaven we have been visiting within ourselves is actually everywhere, and that the steady improvements we have been experiencing in our daily life have been a simple manifestation of this fact. Maybe we did not realize it for quite a long time. Life just got steadily better as we continued with our practices. But then it hits us – the reason for things getting better in daily life is because, not only are we directly perceiving the unbounded realms of peace and joy within us, we are also perceiving them increasingly all around us at the same time.

So, what is within us is also everywhere around us. By going within ourselves during our daily practices, we are also going within everything. By the process of expansion of inner stillness and ecstatic radiance we come to consciously know ourselves to be the essence and substance of every atom of the cosmos.

Thus, we come to know that our existence is cosmic – all-encompassing. Not primarily in an intellectual way, but as a direct experience. How does this happen?

The Marriage of Opposites

We have been focused in this book on developing a reliable practice of spinal breathing pranayama. It is so important to ensure that purification and opening of our nervous system will be progressive and balanced. Spinal breathing also sets the stage for deep meditation, which we have not talked about much here, but is the subject of other AYP writings. We will give it some more attention now, because, while the practices of pranayama and meditation should remain in sequence and separate, it is not possible to separate the relationship of the effects of these two vital methods of spiritual unfoldment.

Spinal breathing is useful for many things. But most of all it is for purifying and opening our spinal nerve and entire nervous system to the flow of ecstatic energy within us. Not that we will experience this on the first day of our practice. But, in time, the necessary openings will occur and we will come to know ecstatic conductivity, and all that comes with it.

Deep meditation cultivates inner silence, which is also called *pure bliss consciousness*. The quality of inner silence is very deep in our nervous system, beyond the flow of ecstatic energy.

Ecstasy is a dynamic quality characterized by movement that can be readily observed in our nervous system once the necessary inner openings have occurred. Bliss is a quality of inner silence and is not dynamic. At least by itself it is not. By itself, the bliss of inner silence can be said to be a self-contained and eternal state of happiness residing deep within us.

With both pranayama and meditation in our twice-daily routine of sitting practices, we are cultivating ecstatic conductivity (ecstasy) and inner silence (bliss) at the same time. One is active and moving around all the time – wanting to radiate. The other is pure awareness, content within itself, a silent witness to all that we experience. These two qualities are opposites.

Along the way, as we are developing these two qualities within us, a remarkable thing happens. There is a merging of the two – a marriage of opposites within us. It is not an instant marriage though. It is one that is occurring over many months and years as we advance along our path of purification and opening. The union is achieved as our ecstatic conductivity and inner silence gradually mature within us. As they do, we find that our ecstatic flow contains more stillness and is more blissful, and that our inner silence becomes more dynamic and is more ecstatic.

Our ecstasy becomes more blissful and our bliss becomes more ecstatic. Then we have to ask ourselves if these two qualities of ecstasy and bliss are still two, or have they become one?

Ecstatic Bliss

If we imagine that there is a border between our unmoving blissful inner silence and the constant movement of ecstatic energy inherent in our rising ecstatic conductivity, how might the marriage of these two qualities occur across this border? It is the classic question of the coexistence of diversity and unity.

How does the One express the many, and how do the many express the One? Well, we may never know intellectually how this happens. But we can surely verify that it does happen in both directions simply by observing from the vantage-point of our inner silence that there is diversity within us and all around us. As we continue with our practices over time, we can also observe the union of our diverse ecstatic flow with our blissful inner silence. If there is a border between ecstasy and bliss, it is dissolved by the process of our purification and opening. Perhaps the border is found only in the obstructions we have been dissolving in our nervous system with the practices of spinal breathing pranayama and deep meditation. Once the obstructions are substantially reduced, then ecstatic conductivity and inner silence merge to become one. This can be called the state of *ecstatic bliss*.

Is this the end? No, it is a new beginning. Now we will consider what this merging of our inner experiences of ecstasy and bliss means on a broader scale.

We have discussed the *radiant* aspect of our experience of ecstatic conductivity, and how this can be both an invisible radiance of energy and also manifested in the form of physical acts containing love and compassion. Where does this love and compassion come from? Is ecstatic energy flow and radiance loving and compassionate? It can be if it is imbued with the deepest qualities of our inner silence. When joined together over time, the qualities of ecstatic energy flow and unmoving inner silence produce a new dynamic containing both movement and the divine attributes of inner silence. This combination of dynamic movement with divine attributes can be called a divine flow, or an outpouring divine love.

The Infinite Self and Divine Love

The beauty of using the simple and highly effective practice of spinal breathing pranayama is that, whether or not we understand the details of the transformation taking place as a result, the process will occur. So, in a way, all of this talk about the marriage of ecstatic conductivity and inner silence, and the rise of outpouring divine love, is a moot point. If the tree is properly fertilized and watered, the fruit will come out. It will happen regardless of any other assessments.

Nevertheless, it is nice to have an idea about where we are going with all of this. Until it happens, the discussion on the ultimate consequences of our practice is merely information – a roadmap. It is good to have a vision of our possibilities. We can then have some benchmarks and be able to verify for ourselves the "cause and effect" of what we are doing. This can inspire us to keep up our daily practice – daily practice over the long term is essential if we are going to proceed smoothly and steadily along our path.

It was mentioned that what we are cultivating within ourselves eventually becomes apparent in our daily surroundings also. In deep meditation we will find the rise of inner silence, which increasingly we come to regard as the center of our sense of self. As this intimate stillness (pure bliss consciousness) within us becomes dynamic through the blending with ecstatic conductivity that is radiating outward into our surrounding environment, then we find that our sense of self moves outward also. In the beginning, we may experience our inner silence as an inactive *witness*, where we find ourselves observing events as though separate from them. This witness, separated from events, is a common experience that arises in those doing deep mediation alone. But when this unmoving witness quality is combined with the rise of ecstatic conductivity, then stillness becomes dynamic in our external environment. Inner silence then combines with the dynamics of everything going on around us. It is an extension of the marriage of opposites within us. Only now it is occurring all around us as well!

What are the implications of this? Quite simply, we find our sense of self emerging everywhere in our daily life. Does this mean we can no longer distinguish our body from that of another? No. It only means that we are able to see oneness, our oneness, and the diversity of our environment at the same time. Then we begin to see by direct perception that our self is truly infinite.

This is not an extension of the ego-self. Rather, it is a dissolving of it. Ego is found in the perception of separateness. In the flowering of enlightenment, this narrow perception gives way to a much greater one – the direct recognition of the omnipresence of our inner silence, and its essential role in the dynamic play of life everywhere.

It is through the practice of spinal breathing pranayama, and its impact on our inner silence cultivated in deep meditation, that this dynamic aspect of perception is activated. It is similar to how we initially entered inner space within our body through the purification and opening of the spinal nerve. From there our experience moves out through every nerve in our body. Then we see the true nature of our inner realms. Similarly, this radiation continues outward until we can see our true nature in everything in our external environment.

The end result of this process is an outpouring of love, compassion and service to others. When enabled by the flow of ecstatic conductivity, inner silence flows out to everyone and everything around us in an effortless embrace. It is natural enough – if we are filled with ecstatic bliss inside, we will also become filled with ecstatic bliss outside. This is the quality that has been observed in the great sages and teachers of all the world's cultures and religions. It is the birthright of every human being.

Spinal breathing pranayama is one of the key practices for activating the profound potential for good that exists within all of us. By taking full advantage of our inner capabilities, we can help ourselves and everyone on the earth move steadily along toward spiritual fulfillment. This is the natural expansion of what we are in our essential nature – divine love.

Further Reading and Support

Yogani is an American spiritual scientist who, for more than thirty years, has been integrating ancient techniques from around the world which cultivate human spiritual transformation. The approach he has developed is non-sectarian, and open to all. In the order published, his books include:

Advanced Yoga Practices – Easy Lessons for Ecstatic Living
A large user-friendly textbook providing 240 detailed lessons on the AYP integrated system of yoga practices.

The Secrets of Wilder – A Novel
The story of young Americans discovering and utilizing actual secret practices leading to human spiritual transformation.

The AYP Enlightenment Series
Easy-to-read instruction books on yoga practices, including:

Deep Meditation – Pathway to Personal Freedom

Spinal Breathing Pranayama – Journey to Inner Space

Tantra – Discovering the Power of Pre-Orgasmic Sex

Asanas, Mudras and Bandhas – Secrets of Inner Ecstasy
(Due out second half 2006)

Samyama – Manifesting the Power of Inner Silence
(Due out second half 2006)

Additional *AYP Enlightenment Series* books are planned…

For up-to-date information on the writings of Yogani, and for the free *AYP Support Forums*, please visit:

www.advancedyogapractices.com

CPSIA information can be obtained at www.ICGtesting.com
Printed in the USA
240404LV00001B/5/A